PSYCHIATRY - THEORY, APPLICATIONS AND TREATMENTS

AF764597

ANTIDEPRESSANTS THERAPY AND RISK OF SUICIDE AMONG PATIENTS WITH MAJOR DEPRESSIVE DISORDERS

Psychiatry - Theory, Applications and Treatments

Additional books in this series can be found on Nova's website under the Series tab.

Additional E-books in this series can be found on Nova's website under the E-book tab.

Pharmacology - Research, Safety Testing and Regulation

Additional books in this series can be found on Nova's website under the Series tab.

Additional E-books in this series can be found on Nova's website under the E-book tab.

PSYCHIATRY - THEORY, APPLICATIONS AND TREATMENTS

ANTIDEPRESSANTS THERAPY AND RISK OF SUICIDE AMONG PATIENTS WITH MAJOR DEPRESSIVE DISORDERS

MAURIZIO POMPILI
PAOLO GIRARDI
DAVID LESTER
AND
ROBERTO TATARELLI

Nova Biomedical Books
New York

Copyright © 2011 by Nova Science Publishers, Inc.

All rights reserved. No part of this book may be reproduced, stored in a retrieval system or transmitted in any form or by any means: electronic, electrostatic, magnetic, tape, mechanical photocopying, recording or otherwise without the written permission of the Publisher.

For permission to use material from this book please contact us:
Telephone 631-231-7269; Fax 631-231-8175
Web Site: http://www.novapublishers.com

NOTICE TO THE READER

The Publisher has taken reasonable care in the preparation of this book, but makes no expressed or implied warranty of any kind and assumes no responsibility for any errors or omissions. No liability is assumed for incidental or consequential damages in connection with or arising out of information contained in this book. The Publisher shall not be liable for any special, consequential, or exemplary damages resulting, in whole or in part, from the readers' use of, or reliance upon, this material. Any parts of this book based on government reports are so indicated and copyright is claimed for those parts to the extent applicable to compilations of such works.

Independent verification should be sought for any data, advice or recommendations contained in this book. In addition, no responsibility is assumed by the publisher for any injury and/or damage to persons or property arising from any methods, products, instructions, ideas or otherwise contained in this publication.

This publication is designed to provide accurate and authoritative information with regard to the subject matter covered herein. It is sold with the clear understanding that the Publisher is not engaged in rendering legal or any other professional services. If legal or any other expert assistance is required, the services of a competent person should be sought. FROM A DECLARATION OF PARTICIPANTS JOINTLY ADOPTED BY A COMMITTEE OF THE AMERICAN BAR ASSOCIATION AND A COMMITTEE OF PUBLISHERS.

Additional color graphics may be available in the e-book version of this book.

Library of Congress Cataloging-in-Publication Data

Antidepressants therapy and risk of suicide among patients with major depressive disorders / Maurizio Pompili ... [et al.].
p. ; cm.
Includes bibliographical references and index.
ISBN 978-1-61728-378-9 (softcover)
1. Suicide--Risk factors. 2. Suicidal behavior--Etiology. 3. Antidepressants--Side effects. 4. Depression, Mental--Treatment--Complications. I. Pompili, Maurizio.
[DNLM: 1. Suicide--psychology. 2. Antidepressive Agents--adverse effects. 3. Depressive Disorder, Major--complications. 4. Depressive Disorder, Major--drug therapy. 5. Risk Assessment. 6. Self-Injurious Behavior--chemically induced. WM 165]
RC569.A75 2010
616.85'8445--dc22

2010035918

Published by Nova Science Publishers, Inc. † New York

Contents

Preface

Most cases of suicide (81%–95%) in the general population involve psychiatric illnesses, nearly half of which (48.5%) are mood disorders. Internationally, the overall average suicide rate has been rising gradually over the past half-century, with increases reported in about half of the nations, mainly among men, and moderate decreases found in the other half, including Northern Europe and North America. This book reviews whether the use of antidepressants is associated with benefits in terms of completed and attempted suicide and whether the increasing use of SSRIs is associated with benefits in terms of decreased rates of suicide, with the aim of generating evidence-based suggestions for clinicians.

Chapter I

Introduction: The Complex Challenge of Suicide

The world-wide annual suicide rate currently averages approximately 13/100,000 (0.013%/year), with higher average rates for men than for women in almost all countries, low rates in children, and relatively high rates in elderly men [1, 2, 3, 4]. Suicide rates vary markedly among regions of the world, countries, and locales, in part reflecting differences in case-identification and reporting procedures [2, 5].

Estimated rates of attempted suicide are much less reliable than rates of completed suicides. Rates of attempted suicide average 20–30 times higher than rates of completed suicide in the general population, but are probably under-reported, and range widely in method and seriousness of intent [6, 7]. The ratio of attempts/suicides in clinical samples of mood-disorder patients is much lower, suggesting a greater lethality of suicidal behaviors [8]. Most cases of suicide (81%–95%) in the general population involve psychiatric illnesses, nearly half of which (48.5%) are mood disorders [9].

Internationally, the overall average suicide rate has been rising gradually over the past half-century, with increases reported in about half of the nations, mainly among men, and moderate decreases found in the other half, including Northern Europe and North America. These improvements could reflect improved diagnosis and treatment of mood disorders during the same era [4, 10, 11, 12, 13].

The risk of completed suicide in patients with mood disorders within five years is two times high in men than in women (8.3% vs. 4.3%), as expected, and most occurred within a year of follow-up after discharge from a psychiatric hospital [14]. The ratio of attempts to subsequent suicides (A/S) is half as great in men as in women (12:1 vs. 23:1), consistent with the greater lethality of suicide attempts in men. The risk of subsequent suicide was higher in men below the age of 35 versus men above the age of 35 (9.7% vs. 7.0%), but higher in women older than this age than those below this age (6.0% vs. 2.5%). Accordingly, the relative risk among younger men was four-times higher than in younger women (9.7% versus 2.5%), whereas the relative risk in older men and women did not differ much (7.0% versus 6.0%), indicating that the lethality of suicidal behavior in women over age 35 approaches that of men of similar age.

Suicide rates are surprisingly high among persons diagnosed with anxiety disorders [15, 16], and severe anxiety may accompany suicidal behavior [17]. Unfortunately, the evidence that anti-anxiety medications reduce suicidal risk in anxiety disorder patients is very limited [16].

The general risk factors for suicide include the presence of a major mood disorder, along with hopelessness, especially when co-occurring with alcohol or substance abuse [2, 6, 9, 18]. The risk is especially high among young adults, impulsive-aggressive individuals and older unmarried men [2, 3]. The risk of suicide in bipolar patients continues to be high despite the introduction of a growing number of new treatments.

Tondo, Lepri, and Baldessarini [19] suggested that the risk of dying by suicide in bipolar disorder patients is nearly 10%, assuming potential risk-exposures of 60 years or more. More than one-third of all suicidal acts occurred within the first year after the onset of the illness, and more than half within the first five years of illness, indicating the need for early diagnosis and intervention for patients with major mood disorders.

Approximately three-quarters of the high proportion of unresolved morbidity among bipolar disorder patients involves depression [20, 21, 22, 23], and this, no doubt, encourages high rates of utilization of antidepressants as a treatment option, even though such treatment is neither approved by regulatory bodies nor well supported by available clinical research as either effective or safe in bipolar patients [24, 25]. Furthermore, antidepressant treatments are associated in some patients with dysphoric-mixed-agitated or psychotic states that can increase the risk of suicidal [26, 27, 28].

The effects of treatments on suicidal risk have been a topic of growing research interest in recent years, but the evidence that most modern psychiatric treatments reduce long-term suicide risks is very limited [2, 3, 29, 30, 31].

In view of this gap, the present book will systematically review whether the use of antidepressants is associated with benefits in terms of completed or attempted suicide and whether the increasing use of SSRIs is associated with benefits in terms of decreased rates of suicide, with the aim of generating evidence-based suggestions for clinicians.

Chapter II

Antidepressants and Suicidal Risk

Only recently have the effects of antidepressant treatments on suicidal behavior and the increased overall mortality associated with major psychiatric disorders become a focus of research interest [32, 33, 34]. A highly controversial question is whether antidepressant treatment modifies the risk of various aspects of "suicidality" among patients with major depressive disorders [35, 36, 37, 38, 39, 40, 41], especially whether the selective serotonin reuptake inhibitors (SSRIs) may cause worsening of suicidal thoughts in vulnerable people [42, 43]. In 2005, a systematic review of published randomized controlled trials comparing SSRIs with other active treatments or placebo found an almost 2-fold increase in the odds of fatal and nonfatal suicide acts among those exposed to SSRIs [44]. However, no increase in risk was observed when only fatal suicide acts were included. Another systematic review by Gunnell et al. [45] compared the use of SSRIs and placebo in adults with depression and other clinical conditions and showed no evidence of increased risk of completed suicide and only weak evidence of increased risk of non-fatal self-harm. More recently, the US Food and Drug Administration (FDA) performed a meta-analysis of individual patient data from 372 randomized placebo-controlled trials of antidepressants, involving a total of nearly 100,000 patients, which concluded that the risk of suicidal behavior was strongly related to age [46]. The risk associated with antidepressant use relative to placebo was increased among patients aged 25 or younger whereas it was reduced among patients aged 65 or older. The overall risk among adult patients aged 25–64 years was not affected, but it was reduced when suicidal ideation and behavior were considered together [47]. Based on these findings, the FDA in 2007 ordered that all antidepressant drugs carry an expanded black-box warning on their label that included information about the increased risk of suicidal behavior in young adults aged 18–24 years [48, 49].

One important limitation to take into account is that the trials included by the FDA were not primarily designed to measure lethal suicidality [47]. (Instead they included a composite outcome of suicide ideas, preparatory acts, andsuicide attempts as well as deaths by suicide.). Additionally, of all suicidal events that were reported, less than 30% were serious suicide attempts or deaths. Also, considering that suicidality was self-reported rather than observed by others in the majority of the clinical trials, it is possible that antidepressant treatment, particularly in younger subjects, may have enhanced communication about suicidality, which may promote more articulated and open thoughts and behaviors.

However, regulatory authorities have issued worldwide warnings about the use of these agents for children and adolescents. The European Medicines Agency (EMEA) has ruled that SSRIs and selective serotonin and norepinephrine reuptake inhibitors (SNRIs) should not be prescribed for depression in children and adolescents under the age of 18. The Committee for the Safety of Medicines in the UK has advised that the balance of risks and benefits for the treatment of depression in the pediatric population is unfavorable for most SSRIs such as paroxetine, citalopram, sertraline, venlafaxine, escitalopram, and mirtazapine. The regulatory authority in the USA requires a safety warning in bold text about suicide risk in package inserts for all antidepressant drugs.

Despite the controversial point of view about the risk of suicide in younger patients, no current evidence indicates a causal relationship between SSRIs and increased risk for suicide in adults. In recent years, many different studies have been performed to explore this issue, including randomized clinical trials, observational studies, case-control studies and ecological analyses.

Among adolescents, a recent study found that SSRI utilization significantly increased the risk of completed or attempted suicide [50] whereas among adults, SSRI use significantly decreased the risk of completed or attempted suicide. Among people aged 65 or more years, the use of SSRIs had a significant protective effect [50]. Among adolescents, exposure to paroxetine and venlafaxine were significantly associated with an increased risk [51, 52], and so the authors directly stated that the effect of age is critical

[50]. However, it is important to note that SSRI treatment was associated with a strong protective effect against depression in all subjects [50].

Finally, it is important to note that the majority of studies on the effect of antidepressant therapy on the risk of suicide have a number of limitations. First, observational studies have limited ability to adjust for baseline differences and are prone to bias and confounding. Also, among adolescents, SSRI treatment is often reserved for very severe cases, and so the higher suicide rate might be confounded by severity, that is, adolescents who received SSRIs might have been more severely depressed (and more suicidal) than adolescents who did not receive SSRIs. In contrast, among adults, SSRIs may be prescribed similarly in very severe and less severe cases, and confounding may be less important. Only a few of the studies considered confounding factors such as the different severity of the illness for which the antidepressant medication was prescribed. Olfson et al. [51] limited their analysis to individuals who received inpatient treatment for depression, thereby ensuring a fairly comparable level of illness severity. In two other studies, comparability between groups was increased by the comparison of the risk of suicide during SSRI use with the risk during no antidepressant use in the same cohort [52, 53].

Barbui et al [50] noted that, athough re-analyses of randomized studies, including the FDA study, reported similar differences between antidepressants [49, 54, 55], it is not clear why the use of some antidepressants, such as paroxetine and venlafaxine, increases the risk of suicide more than the use of other antidepressants. New evidence, such as head-to-head comparisons, are needed to test the long-term efficacy and safety of these medication in clinical practice, particularly in younger patients. A very close monitoring is suggested for children and adolescents who are prescribed antidepressants for the possibility of an increased risk of suicidal thoughts or suicidal behaviors.

Chapter III

The Relationship between Antidepressants and Suicide as Reported in Ecological Studies

As we have seen, the evidence that antidepressant treatment yields expected reductions in the risk of suicides or attempts is controversial. Several studies suggest that, in most of the Nordic countries and in the USA, the emergence of modern antidepressants over the past decade in current clinical practice has been associated with generally moderate decreases in overall suicide rates, varying by sex and age groups [10, 11, 13, 56, 57, 58, 59, 60, 61, 62, 63]. However, in the USA and some Nordic countries, similar trends involving a reduction in suicide rates were also reported a decade before the introduction of fluoxetine, the first clinically successful modern antidepressant [13, 63].

Recently Baldessarini et al. [13] found that only nine of 29 ecological studies reported significant inverse correlations between increased use of modern antidepressants and declining trends in suicide rates. Another six found no relationships and 14 found correlations in some sex or age subgroups that were inconsistent across studies.

Also, data from 78 reporting countries indicated that only about half of the nations (54%) experienced decreases in annual suicide rates between the 1950s (when antidepressants were not available) and the early 2000s (a decade after introduction of modern antidepressants) and, in contrast, a similar proportion (46%) reported increases in suicide rates. Similar decreases and increases were reported in the separate regions of Western and Eastern Europe, Latin America and Asia. The World Health Organization has concluded that the distribution of decreases and increases in the suicide rates of nations between 1990 and the early 2000s was similar [4]. These data suggest the existence of a highly complex phenomenon which reflects the existence of many contributing factors.

Ecological studies should be considered in the light of several limitations. First, it is possible that improvements in public health, changes in legal, cultural or social prohibitions against suicide, and improvements in identifying and reporting suicides might be associated with higher suicide rates despite the increased access to modern psychopharmacological treatment in the majority of countries. Socioeconomic factors may also contribute to the complex findings from the ecological studies as well as access to clinical services and social support. Finally, all correlational studies suffer from a fundamental inability to relate medication exposure or other specific factors *causally* to suicidal behavior at the level of individuals [64].

Our concludion is that ecological studies cannot prove a direct, causal relationship between antidepressant treatment and reduced suicidal risk at the level of individual persons, and further research with less ambiguous methods is needed.

Chapter IV

The Relationship between Antidepressants and Suicide as Reported in Cohort and Case-Control Studies

Data from cohort and case-control studies suggest that the utilization of antidepressants markedly increased during the 1990s, but in recent years has partially decreased as a result of concerns regarding the emergence of suicidality during antidepressant treatment.

Bailly [65] suggested that, relative to placebo, SSRIs are efficacious for pediatric cases of affective disorder but may be associated with a modest increase in the risk of suicidal ideation and behavior. Bailly reported that the use of SSRIs is also associated with a significant decrease in the suicide rates of children and adolescents, presumably because of the efficacy of SSRIs, the compliance of the patients, and the low toxicity in overdose. Recent research suggests that antidepressants may be protective against early readmission after hospitalization for suicide attempts or ideation [66]. These data, taken together, indicate that SSRIs can improve adolescent depression better than placebo [67], although the magnitude of the antidepressant effect is only small to moderate because of a high placebo response.

Recent attention and wide-scale interventions by regulatory authorities have changed drug usage patterns. In a 9-year cohort study of 20,906 children who began antidepressant therapy, Schneeweiss et al. [68] found that 266 children attempted suicide and three completed suicide, with no meaningful differences in the rate s when comparing various SSRIs. They supported the decision of the Food and Drug Administration to include all antidepressants in the black box warning regarding the potentially increased risk of suicidal behavior for children and adolescents who begin the use of antidepressants.

The same authors [68] suggested that treatment decisions should be based on efficacy, and clinicians should be vigilant in monitoring patients after initiating therapy with any antidepressant. In a cohort study of 287,543 adults aged 18 years and older who were users of antidepressants, they found that most events occurred in the first six months after the initiation of treatment and that there was no clinically meaningful variation in the risk of suicide and suicide attempt between the antidepressants.

However, the possible relationship between psychotropic pharmacotherapy and suicidal behavior among children and adolescents remains unclear. The increased risk of suicidality in adolescents, compared to adults, is weak but consistent across most studies, although epidemiological studies do not support a clear relationship between use of antidepressants and the completed suicide rate [67].

Reeves and Ladner [69] suggested that antidepressant-induced suicidality is an uncommon occurrence but also a legitimate phenomenon. Close monitoring is needed, and adequate follow-up care should be provided for patients after the initiation of a new antidepressant.

Other sources of data about this controversial topic include large cohorts of depressed patients from general practice or health-maintenance organization data sources, and relatively large, case-control comparisons of subgroups varying in exposure to antidepressants. Such studies include over one million, mainly clinically depressed subjects in 17 reports [51, 52, 70, 71, 72, 73, 74, 75, 76, 77, 78, 79, 80, 81, 82, 83, 84]. These studies have yielded inconsistent findings. Many (n=11) were designed to test for greater suicidal risk with SSRIs compared to other agents or to non-treatment. Nine of these 11 studies did not find evidence of greater suicidal risk associated with antidepressant treatment. A majority of the remaining studies (4 out of the 6) found a decreased or no difference in suicidal risk with more antidepressant treatment.

A few of these studies found greater suicidal risk with more antidepressant treatment in general or, specifically, with the greater use of SSRIs and other modern antidepressants, in particular, small increases among adolescents [51, 84], larger increases in elderly patients [81], as well as fewer completed suicides but more attempts [52].

However, data from these studies are severely compromised by the risk of confounding by morbidity or by indication. Medical treatments, in general, are more likely to be given to more severely ill patients at a higher risk of suicide, and treatment with a low risk of toxic effects from acute overdosing (such as the SSRIs) is more likely to be selected clinically than treatment with more toxic agents (such as the tricyclic antidepressants) for patients at increased risk for suicide. Additionally, the nonrandomized, clinically-selected treatment in such studies may severely distort the associations observed between greater suicidal risk and the use of some treatments.

Chapter V

The Relationship between Antidepressants and Suicide as Reported in Randomized Controlled Trials (RCTs)

RCTs should be the most reliable source of data on the effects of antidepressant treatment on suicidal risk. Individual trials are unlikely to include enough patients with identified suicidal acts to allow testing for treatment effects, especially since being acutely suicidal is usually a criterion for exclusion from such trials. However, meta-analytic methods may yield substantial numbers of suicide attempts and even completed suicides.

Rates of suicide attempts, and even of completed suicides, may be as high in controlled trials as in clinical samples of patients with major depressive disorder. Suicide rates taken from large meta-analyses of modern and older antidepressants or placebo (given similar rates with all treatments) averaged 862/100,000/year [85, 86, 87], or 66-times above the average international general population suicide rate of 13/100,000/year [4]. In clinical samples of severely ill patients with major depressions, usually hospitalized patients, the standardized mortality ratio (SMR) for suicide compared to the general population was 20-times higher [15], and among less severely ill, depressed patients the SMR may be about three-times higher [88]. Such high observed rates of suicidal behaviors in RCTs reflect exaggeration arising from annualizing rates based on relatively brief exposure times (typically 8–12 weeks) in most trials involving patients with acute depression, early in the course of treatment.

There have been several recent reports, based on pooled data, on rates of suicides and suicide attempts from large numbers of RCTs and subjects and involving modern antidepressants, older standard agents and placebo [37, 44, 45, 47, 85, 86, 87, 89, 90, 91, 92, 93]. With the exception of one report which found a significant excess of suicidal acts during treatment with SSRIs [44], other meta-analyses have found only minor differences in the rates of suicidal behaviors between depressed patients treated with an SSRI, other antidepressants, or a placebo, tending overall toward an apparently greater risk with antidepressants. It was assumed that the trials included in the meta-analyses were well-randomized and with well-balanced exposures in both the drug and placebo arms throughout the duration of the trials.

Baldessarini et al. [37] reported in a meta-analysis that the overall pooled Rate Ratio (RR) was 1.42, compared to the null value of RR=1.0 whereas Fergusson et al. [44] reported a relatively large RR. The authors concluded that more than 600 depressed patients would have to be exposed to an antidepressant drug for approximately two months (or about 100 treated for a year), early in the course of an episode of an acute major depressive disorder, when the suicidal risk is particularly high, to yield one excess suicide attempt, and over 4,500 depressed patients to yield one excess suicide over the number associated with untreated major depression.

An FDA review [47] analyzed all available data from 386 controlled trials of modern antidepressant drugs involving 112,875 patients with major depressive or other disorders. Most of the identified suicidal events involved suicidal ideation, but they were of uncertain clinical significance. Reported instances of suicides (0.013%) and attempts (0.198%) may have been low due to the relatively brief exposure times, which averaged only two months. Among adult patients diagnosed with a major depressive disorder, the observed suicide rate, based on estimated exposure-times averaging eight weeks, was 77/100,000/year, or only six-times above the general population rate of 13/100,000/year [4], compared to suicide rates of 862/100,000/year found in similar controlled trials of modern antidepressants, as already noted [85, 86, 87]. Stratifying by age-groups suggested an increased risk of broadly defined "suicidality" (mainly ideation) with modern antidepressants versus placebo at younger ages and possible beneficial effects in older patients. It is important to note that, based on these data, completed suicide and attempted suicide were rare.

These findings suggest an increased risk of presumably new suicidal ideation with SSRIs and other modern antidepressants over placebo among children, adolescents and young adults up to age 24 years and extended the initial impressions of a similar finding in meta-analyses involving children and adolescents by the UK drug regulatory agency [94] and the FDA [91, 93].

However, RCTs should be considered according to the following limitations. First, the data fail to support an expected overall reduction in the risk of suicidal acts during treatment with antidepressants of all types and suggest that the risk of suicide attempts and perhaps completed suicides may be greater during treatment with certain antidepressants. Furthermore, although many trials involving patients with depressive disorder found substantially larger reductions in average ratings of suicidal ideation with antidepressants of various types than with placebo [87, 89, 95, 96, 97], unfortunately these trials reported subjective data, usually incidental, and based on post-hoc assessments of individual items on standard depression symptom-rating scales (Hamilton item 3 or Montgomery-Åsberg item 10).

Additionally, these RCTs are limited by the potential unreliability of essentially incidental, passive reporting of suicidal thoughts or behaviors based on currently typical “adverse event reporting” systems. The relatively short duration of most trials of treatments for acute depression may not provide an adequate evaluation of the effects of treatment on rare suicidal behaviors, comparable to the long-term trials available for clozapine, lithium and anticonvulsants. Another potential source of bias is that the initial randomization in RCTs can break down during the conduct of trials. Premature, and potentially non-random, dropping out, usually a result of the lack of any perceived benefit or the emergence of intolerable side effects of the treatment, is routinely found in most RCTs. Observed rates of “suicidal events” are rarely corrected for the actual time of exposure of individual patients to specific treatments. Such a correction for actual adverse event rates (events/persons/weeks) may be important if actual exposures are not closely matched across the trial treatment arms, particularly when rare events such as completed and attempted suicides are involved [98].

After considering all the data, the FDA demanded warnings about the possible increased of risk of suicidal ideation and perhaps behaviors during the treatment of juvenile and young adult patients with SSRIs and other modern antidepressants. This decision was based on at least four controlled trials [99], one of which was a very large federally-funded trial with an unusually large separation of responses to the drug versus placebo [100]. In 12 relatively large trials of SSRIs in juvenile patients with major depression, the relative rate of responding to the drug relative to the placebo (RR) averaged 1.23 and in 14 much smaller trials of TCAs, the pooled RR of 1.15 was of similarly modest magnitude but statistically nonsignificant [99]. The conclusion about the possible worsening of suicidality in young antidepressant-treated patients is that there are clinical developmental differences in affective and behavioral responses to antidepressants that require further study, especially with respect to the risk of actual suicidal behaviors.

Chapter VI

The Relationship between Antidepressants and Suicide in Different Countries

In recent years, antidepressant prescribing has increased markedly in many developed countries, especially after the introduction of the SSRIs in the early 1990s. This might reflect the better recognition, treatment and prescribing for depression and also the advantage that lethal overdoses of these new medications are rare. The associations between antidepressants and suicide rates differ by country. In Italy, Barbui et al. [101] described the impact of regulatory changes on antidepressant consumption in Italy from 1988 to 1996, examining whether the introduction of SSRIs was associated with changes in overall suicide rates [101]. Data on suicide, available from 1988 to 1994, showed that, in the seven-year period during which SSRI use rose, male suicide rates increased from 9.8 to 10.2 per 100,000 inhabitants and females suicide rates declined from 3.9 to 3.2 per 100,000 inhabitants. The authors concluded that, in Italy, there was not any dramatic reduction in the overall suicide rates as a result of the increasing prescribing of SSRIs. Guaiana et al. [102], investigating the impact of the increasing use of SSRIs and newer antidepressants on suicide rates, reported that, in Italy from 1983 to 2000, the use of tricyclic antidepressants remained stable and the use of SSRIs and newer agents dramatically increased. Suicide rates for males decreased from 1955 to 1974 and subsequently increased, reaching a peak in 1985, and then declined. In females, suicide rates remained substantially stable until 1978. Suicide by poisoning dropped by nearly 50% from 1986 to 2000. Long-term analysis did not indicate that the increase in antidepressant prescribing was accompanied by a reduction in the suicide rate. In Italy, newer antidepressants had no impact on the total number of admissions for depression, nor on the proportion of all admissions.

In Sweden, Carlsten et al. [103] performed a time-series analysis using a two-slope model to compare suicide rates before and after the introduction of the SSRIs. Antidepressant sales increased in men from 4.2 DDD/1,000 inhabitants/day during 1977-1979 to 21.8 in 1995-1997, and in women from 8.8 to 42.4 DDD/1,000 inhabitants/day between the same periods. A particularly rapid acceleration in antidepressant sales was observed during the years 1993-1996. In the two census periods, suicide rates decreased in men by 30.9% and in women by 34.0%. The slope of suicide rates significantly changed after 1990, corresponding to 348 fewer suicides than expected during 1990-1997. This study showed a statistically significant change in the slope in suicide rates among men and women that coincided with the introduction of the SSRIs in Sweden. However, the advent of SSRIs may explain only part of the declining suicide trend, because this trend started years before these drugs were introduced. Isacsson [10] found that suicide rate decreased by 19% in parallel with the increased use of antidepressants in Sweden, Denmark, Norway and Finland. Moreover, in Sweden there was no demographic group with regard to age, gender or county in which the suicide rate decreased in the absence of an increased use of antidepressants. Thus, the author concluded that the increased use of antidepressants appeared to be one of the contributing factors to the decrease in the suicide rate. Ohberg et al. [104] found that, in Finland from 1990 to 1995, the total suicide rate decreased from 30.3 per 100,000 inhabitants to 27.2. The total consumption of antidepressants more than doubled from 1990 to 1995. The authors concluded that the increased use of SSRIs in Finland coincided with a significant decline in suicide mortality. However, suicides using antidepressants showed an upward trend.

Rihmer reported that, in Hungary, in which suicide was an alarming phenomenon, the suicide rate steadily declined from 45.9 per 100,000 inhabitants in 1984 to 32.1 in 1998 [105, 106, 107]. This decrease occurred together with the implementation of a new system of psychiatric care in which the number of outpatient psychiatric departments increased between 1982 and 1998, the number of psychiatrists increased between 1986 and 1998, and the number of emergency telephone services increased during the same period. Antidepressant consumption, mainly SSRIs, rose from 1984 to 1998 with an approximately fivefold increase. In the same period there was a sixfold increase in unemployment, a 25% rise in official estimates of alcoholism rates and a 21% increase in divorce. The author concluded that suicide rates are affected by many factors, and the association between improved pharmacotherapy for depression and decreased suicide mortality is not easily demonstrated.

Hall and colleagues [108] found that, in Australia between 1991 and 2000, the suicide rate markedly decreased in elderly men and women and increased in young adults especially young men, yielding a stable total suicide rate. Exposure to antidepressants was higher for women than men in all age groups and increased markedly for both men and women, with the largest increases among older adults. A significant negative association was observed between antidepressants consumption and suicide in women but not in men. However, among both men and women, the largest declines in suicide occurred in the age groups with the highest exposure to antidepressants.

Grunebaum et al. [11] reported that, in the United States from 1985 to 1999, the decline in the national suicide rate appeared to be associated with a greater use of non-tricyclic antidepressants. Suicide rates were already declining before 1985 in the United States, especially in females [109, 110]. In an ecological analysis over counties in the USA, Gibbons and colleagues [57] found that the overall association between antidepressant prescriptions and the suicide rate was not significant for prescriptions for SSRIs, but the prescription of other new-generation non-SSRI antidepressants (nefazodone hydrochloride, mirtazapine, bupropion hydrochloride, and venlafaxine hydrochloride) were associated with lower suicide rates (both within and between counties).

Davis et al. [111] studied whether higher suicide risk, defined as previous suicide attempts or suicidal ideation, influenced the choice of antidepressant prescribed in the UK. They found that a risk of suicide did not prevent the prescription of venlafaxine, and that venlafaxine therapy is considered to be acceptable when appropriately managed. Gunnell et al. [112] reported a time-series analysis revealing an increase in young male suicide in England and Wales in the last 30 years in parallel with a rise in a number of risk factors for suicide in this age group. In people aged over 60 an association was found between a decline in suicide and increases in the gross domestic product, antidepressant prescribing and other measures of improved healthcare provision.

In a longitudinal analyses of pooled data from 15 placebo-controlled, randomized, double-blind, short-term trials of mirtazapine conducted in Austria, Kasper et al. [113] found that mirtazapine was associated with a statistically significant lower risk of suicidality compared to placebo.

In the pediatric population, higher SSRI prescription rates were associated with lower suicide rates in children and adolescents [58]. Similar findings were reported by Olfson and colleagues [51] in an extensive analysis of prescription data in the USA. However, all these positive finding may reflect not only the efficacy of SSRIs, but also better compliance by patients, improved quality of mental health care and a low toxicity in the event of a suicide attempt by overdose.

In Northern Ireland, Kelly et al. [114] observed that, in the younger group, there was no association between antidepressant prescribing and suicide while, for the older group, increased antidepressant prescribing was associated with a reduction in suicide rate over a period of 10 years. However, a subsequent analysis of UK data suggested that the decline in suicide rates happened before the increases in prescribing. Moreover, rises in antidepressant prescribing did not consistently coincide with clear changes in suicide trends [115]. Also in England, Morgan et al. [116] investigated mortality from suicide and suggested that the increased prescribing of antidepressants, a proxy measure of improved diagnosis and treatment of depression in primary care, was accompanied by lower suicide rates.

In Iceland sales of antidepressants increased from 1975 to 2000, but suicide rates fluctuated during 1950-2000 and did not show any definite trend [56].

Finally, in Israel, the prescribing of antidepressants, particularly of SSRIs, increased 2.6-fold between 1998 and 2002. An overall reduction in suicides, significant only in elderly men, was reported in association with this increased rate of antidepressant prescription [117].

Chapter VII

Possible Explanations for the Lack of Effect on Suicidal Risk During Antidepressant Treatment and Clinical Implications

Several explanations for the lack of an overall beneficial effect on risk of suicides and suicide attempts during antidepressant treatment have been proposed, including limitations in the clinical effectiveness of antidepressants, particularly in younger age-groups and for some features of depressive illnesses that may be particularly pertinent to suicidal risk, as well as technical limitations of the available studies of antidepressant treatment and suicide [36]. An additional possibility is that antidepressants may have both beneficial and adverse effects, with a net null average impact on suicidal risk.

This is supported by the long tradition of clinical observations, including the proposal that temporal separation of the relatively earlier energizing effects of mood-elevating drugs from the later benefits on the anhedonic features of depression might increase the risk of suicidal behavior during recovery from acute major depressive episodes [118]. Additionally, there are a series of clinical observations of newly emerging aggressive and suicidal preoccupations or behaviors among patients being treated with antidepressants. Whether such reactions may not be more frequent with SSRIs than with older antidepressants such as tricyclics (TCAs) is still unclear.

However, it is well-known that antidepressant treatment is associated in some antidepressant-treated patients with over-stimulation, restlessness resembling akathisia, agitation, insomnia, severe anxiety, mixed-dysphoric bipolar states, and psychosis [119, 120, 121, 122, 123]. Such paradoxical effects of antidepressant treatment have received attention in recent international discussions of risk/benefit considerations arising from studies of SSRIs, particularly for juvenile depressive disorders. These discussions consider the seemingly limited benefits of antidepressant treatment of all types in juvenile depression against the concern about potential increases in suicidality that include the still-uncertain risks of eventual suicide attempts and the very low rates of completed suicides [124].

Table 1. Proposed risk factors and warning signs for emerging suicidality during antidepressant treatment

▪	Previous suicide attempts or violent acts
▪	Known or suspected bipolarity
▪	Severe, recurring depression
▪	Known or suspected psychotic illness
▪	Juvenile depression
▪	Agitation, akathisia, anxiety
▪	Insomnia
▪	Anger, aggression or threats of aggression
▪	Irritable dysphoria
▪	Switching into mixed bipolar or psychotic states
▪	Worsening of depression, hopelessness, anguish
▪	Helplessness or social isolation
▪	Current stressors (loss, separation, scandal, financial crisis)
▪	New somatic symptoms
▪	Abuse of alcohol or other disinhibiting central depressants, including anxiolytics such as benzodiazepines
▪	Ready access to firearms, hoarded drugs or other toxins
▪	Inadequate clinical supervision and follow-up

*Modified from Pompili et al. [130].

The scientific and clinical significance of the effects of antidepressant treatment on suicidal risk requires further critical study, although our clinical impression is that antidepressant treatment may present certain behavioral risks that require close clinical monitoring, ongoing differential clinical assessment, and adequate interventions to optimize the effectiveness and safety of antidepressant treatment.

However, several warning signs including prominent anxiety and irritability, anger, and agitation early in the use of an antidepressant, particularly in antidepressant monotherapy, should be looked for and guide clinicians in treating patients with higher suicidal risk. Those with likely or suspected bipolar features or psychotic illnesses call for particular concern when under antidepressant monotherapy without the presumably protective effects of mood-stabilizing or antipsychotic agents. These and other suggested warning signs or risk factors are summarized in Table 1.

Chapter VIII

Adverse Effect of Antidepressants and Suicide Mortality

In 2004, two systematic reviews about the efficacy and safety data of antidepressants for children and adolescents were simultaneously published, one in the *British Medical Journal* [125] and the other in *Lancet* [124]. Jureidini et al. [125] checked the quality of methods in published trials of antidepressants in children and adolescents in a total of 477 patients from six randomized trials who were treated with paroxetine, fluoxetine, sertraline or venlafaxine and 464 treated with placebo. Of 42 reported outcome measures, only 14 showed a statistical advantage for antidepressant drugs. Regarding the adverse effects of treatment, the authors suggested that some adverse effects might be more frequent than the authors of these studies imply. For example, up to half of young patients experienced an "activation syndrome", and self-injurious ideation was seen in 6% of the patients [126]. However, their analysis did not investigate the relative frequency of this rare outcome. In the second study, Whittington et al. [124] reported no increased risk of suicidal behavior with fluoxetine compared to placebo (3.6% versus 3.8%), but an increased risk of suicidal ideation or attempting suicide was observed for paroxetine (3.7% versus 2.5%), sertraline (2.6% versus 1.2%), citalopram (7.1% versus 3.6%,) and venlafaxine (7.7% versus 0.6%).

Jick and collegues [70] followed 172,598 people who had at least one prescription for one of ten antidepressant drugs in general practice in the UK and found that the risk of suicide was higher in people who received fluoxetine

(19/10,000 person years, 95%CI 9 to 34) than in those receiving dosulepine (dothiepin). In a nested case-controlled subgroup analysis in people with no history of suicidal behavior or previous antidepressant prescription, the risk remained the same, although the confidence interval broadened to make the result nonsignificant. However, they did not report the eventual association between the adverse events in patients taking antidepressants and the risk of completed suicide.

Jick and colleagues [71] performed a matched case-control study of more than 2,500 patients and reported that the risk of suicidal behavior after starting antidepressant treatment was similar among users of amitriptyline, fluoxetine, and paroxetine compared with the risk among users of dothiepin. The risk of suicidal behavior was similar in patients taking SSRIs and tricyclics, but dothiepin might not be a useful comparison antidepressant for countries where this agent has never been licensed, such as Italy and USA [127].

To replicate this finding, Jick et al. [71] used amitriptyline as a reference compound, and the ORs for non-fatal suicidal behaviors among users of the other three antidepressants were 1.21 (0.80-1.83) for dothiepin, 1.40 (0.92-2.13) for fluoxetine and 1.55 (0.99-2.43) for paroxetine. A borderline value for paroxetine in comparison with amitriptyline emerged in this post-hoc analysis, leaving the possibility of an increased risk of non-fatal suicidal behaviors in users of this agent.

To test the potential empirical link between antidepressant treatment and suicide attempts Valuck and colleagues [128] investigated 24,000 adolescents using a community sample of managed-care enrolees in the USA. Crude suicide attempt rates ranged from 0.0% to 2.3% by index treatment group. Treatment with SSRIs (hazard ratio 1.59), other antidepressant drugs (hazard ratio 1.03) or multiple antidepressants (hazard ratio 1.43) resulted in no significant increased risk of a suicide attempt. In contrast, Martinez et al. [79] analyzed the risk of non-fatal self-harm and suicide in 146,095 patients with a new diagnosis of depression who were prescribed SSRIs or tricyclics. SSRI users in comparison with tricyclic users were not at increased risk of suicide or non-fatal self-harm. However, in patients aged 18 or less, weak evidence suggested a higher risk of non-fatal self-harm in those prescribed SSRIs (OR 1.59). Søndergård et al. [84] investigated the association between SSRIs and suicide in children and adolescents in Denmark and observed a statistically nonsignificant increased rate of suicides associated with SSRI use (RR 4.47). Simon et al. [82] identified more than 65,000 individuals with more than 82,000 episodes of antidepressant treatment. The risk of suicide during the acute-phase treatment was one in 3,000 treatment episodes and the risk of a serious suicide attempt was one in 1,000. The data did not indicate a significant increase in the risk of suicide or serious suicide attempt after starting treatment with the newer antidepressants.

Isacsson et al. [61] analyzed the presence of different antidepressants in the forensic toxicological screening of 14,857 suicides compared with those in 26,422 cases of deaths by accident or natural causes in Sweden from 1992 to 2000. In the toxicological screening, antidepressants were detected in 3,096 (20%) of the 14,857 cases of suicide investigated and a total of 3,411 antidepressants were identified in these individuals. Of these, 48% were SSRIs, whereas the number of detections in the 26,422 controls was 1,538 (5.8%). SSRIs were under-represented compared with other antidepressants (OR 0.83). The differences within the SSRIs were nonsignificant, with the exception of fluvoxamine. The OR for the tricyclics as a class (including maprotiline) was 1.01, but it was higher for the class of moclobemide, mianserin, mirtazapine, reboxetine and venlafaxine (OR 1.78, 99%CI 1.46-2.16). In 52 cases of suicide in those aged less than 15 years, seven were positive for antidepressants (clomipramine, imipramine, maprotiline, trimipramine, mianserin and venlafaxine), but no SSRIs were detected. In 326 cases of suicide in the 15 to 19 year-old group, there were 13 cases which were positive for antidepressants (amitriptyline, clomipramine, trimipramine, citalopram, fluoxetine, sertraline and mirtazapine), and SSRIs had a lower RR compared with non-SSRIs. Thus, the hypothesis that treatment of depressed individuals with SSRIs leads to an increased risk of suicide was not supported by this analysis of suicides in Sweden over a period of 9 years.

In a nationwide cohort study in Finland, Tiihonen et al. [52] studied the association between the risk of suicide, attempted suicide, and overall mortality associated with antidepressant use, calculating the RR of completed suicides, suicide attempts leading to hospitalization and overall mortality during tricyclic, SSRI and SNRI treatment versus no antidepressant use, after adjusting for possible confounders. In the entire cohort, fluoxetine use (RR 0.52) was associated with a lower risk of suicide and venlafaxine (RR 1.61) with a higher risk. Among suicidal subjects who had ever used antidepressants, the current use of any antidepressants was associated with a markedly increased risk of attempted suicide and with a markedly decreased risk of completed suicide.

The relationship between venlafaxine use and suicidality was also investigated by Rubino et al. [129] who found that patients prescribed venlafaxine were more likely to complete or attempt suicide compared with patients prescribed citalopram, fluoxetine and dothiepin, but adjustment for a number of possible confounders substantially reduced the excess risk. Finally, Juurlink and colleagues [81] explored the relationship between the initiation of treatment with SSRIs and completed suicide in older patients. During the first month of therapy, SSRI utilization was associated with a nearly fivefold higher risk of completed suicide over the other antidepressants (adjusted odds ratio 4.8). The risk was independent of a recent diagnosis of depression or the receipt of psychiatric care, and suicides of a violent nature were more common during SSRI therapy.

However, the absolute risk of suicide was low, maybe suggesting that the response to these agents may induce suicide only in a specific vulnerable subgroup of patients.

Chapter IX

Conclusion

Research on the possible relationship between pharmacotherapy and suicidal behavior was virtually unknown until a decade ago. An initial case series and several reports, especially in the last ten years, have indicated that a minority of depressed patients experience adverse behavioral and emotional responses to treatment with various antidepressant drugs, including SSRIs [38, 120, 130]. Some ecological studies have reported minor decreases in suicide rates by region or time correlated with higher rates of prescribing modern antidepressants, but such correlations are presumably influenced by many factors associated with access to clinical care. Most large clinical studies indicate decreased suicidal risk with antidepressant treatment but, in contrast, some find increases for patients in some age groups. However, these studies often have confounding variables such as an association between antidepressant treatment and more severe depression and, thus, greater suicidal risk. Data pooled from relatively brief, randomized, controlled trials in patients with acute major depression suggest an increase in the risk of suicide attempts, as well as increases in suicidal ideation in younger patients, but decreases in elderly patients.

These data, taken together, suggest that antidepressants do not always have a beneficial effect on the risk of suicidal behaviors, although they may reduce both suicidal ideation and other depressive symptoms. Peculiar responses, often emerging early in the course of antidepressant treatment, require a close clinical follow-up in order to monitor the suicidal risk. When this kind of risk is identified, treatment should be appropriately modified, for example, by changing the antidepressant medication, adding sedating, antipsychotic or mood-stabilizing treatments, and providing additional individual support.

Suggested pharmacological interventions and other clinical steps aimed at safe management of patients at risk for the types of adverse behavioral responses to antidepressants are summarized in Table 2.

Table 2. Proposed interventions for emerging suicidal risk during antidepressant treatment

▪	Decrease dose, or suspend antidepressant therapy if new agitation, insomnia, or anger emerges
▪	Introduce an atypical antipsychotic, anticonvulsant, or sedative
▪	Consider lithium for cooperative patients, especially following *inadequate* antidepressant responses
▪	Make explicit the collaborative and flexible nature of treatment; emphasize the clinician's availability for extra routine visits or calls, as well as in emergencies
▪	Express explicit concern for growing discomfort and despair
▪	Address suicidality directly and repeatedly, and monitor for access to lethal means of self-injury, including hoarded drugs, other toxins, or firearms
▪	Enlist the help of a family member to monitor the patient and perhaps to dispense medicines

*Modified from Pompili et al. [130].

We may conclude that, in general, antidepressant drugs appear to reduce suicidal ideation in depressed adults. Whether these agents reduce the suicidal risk in younger patients is still a matter of debate.

References

[1] Goldsmith, S.K.; Pellmar, T.C.; Kleinman, A.M.; Bunney, W.E., *Reducing suicide: A national imperative*; Joseph Henry Press: Washington, D.C., 2002.

[2] American Psychiatric Association *Practice guideline for the assessment and treatment of patients with suicidal behaviors*; American Psychiatric Association: Arlington, 2003.

[3] Simon, R.I.; Hales, R.E. *The American Psychiatric Publishing textbook of suicide assessment and management*; American Psychiatric Press: Washington, DC, 2006.

[4] World Health Organization (WHO) International suicide rates. Available online: www.who.int/mental_health/prevention/suicide/country_reports/en/index.html (01/10).

[5] Diekstra, R.F. The epidemiology of suicide and parasuicide. *Acta Psychiatr. Scand. Suppl.* 1993, *371*, 9-20.

[6] Tondo, L.; Isacsson, G.; Baldessarini, R.J. Suicide in bipolar disorder: risk and prevention. *CNS Drugs*. 2003, *17*, 491-511.

[7] Kessler, R.C.; Berglund, P.; Borges, G.; Nock, M.; Wang, P.S. Trends in suicide ideation, plans, gestures, and attempts in the United States, 1990-1992 to 2001-2003. *Jama*. 2005, *293*, 2487-2495.

[8] Baldessarini, R.J.; Tondo, L.; Davis, P.; Pompili, M.; Goodwin, F.K.; Hennen, J. Decreased risk of suicides and attempts during long-term lithium treatment: a meta-analytic review. *Bipolar. Disord.* 2006, *8*, 625-639.

[9] Roy, A. Suicide. In *Kaplan and Sadock's Comprehensive Textbook of Psychiatry, chapter 29.1*; 7th ed.; Sadock, B. J.; Sadock, V. A., Eds.;

Lippincott Willians and Wilkins: Philadelphia, 2000; Vol. 2, pp. 2031–2040.

[10] Isacsson, G. Suicide prevention--a medical breakthrough? *Acta Psychiatr. Scand.* 2000, *102*, 113-117.

[11] Grunebaum, M.F.; Ellis, S.P.; Li, S.; Oquendo, M.A.; Mann, J.J. Antidepressants and suicide risk in the United States, 1985-1999. *J. Clin. Psychiatry.* 2004, *65*, 1456-1462.

[12] Tondo, L.; Baldessarini, R.J. Trends in suicide rates: an international perspective. *Ital. J. Psychopathol.* 2006, *12*, 202-203.

[13] Baldessarini, R.J.; Tondo, L.; Strombom, I.M.; Dominguez, S.; Fawcett, J.; Licinio, J.; Oquendo, M.A.; Tollefson, G.D.; Valuck, R.J.; Tohen, M. Ecological studies of antidepressant treatment and suicidal risks. *Harv. Rev. Psychiatry.* 2007, *15*, 133-145.

[14] Nordstrom, P.; Samuelsson, M.; Asberg, M. Survival analysis of suicide risk after attempted suicide. *Acta Psychiatr. Scand.* 1995, *91*, 336-340.

[15] Harris, E.C.; Barraclough, B. Excess mortality of mental disorder. *Br. J. Psychiatry.* 1998, *173*, 11-53.

[16] Khan, A.; Leventhal, R.M.; Khan, S.; Brown, W.A. Suicide risk in patients with anxiety disorders: a meta-analysis of the FDA database. *J. Affect. Disord.* 2002, *68*, 183-190.

[17] Fawcett, J. Treating impulsivity and anxiety in the suicidal patient. *Ann. N. Y. Acad. Sci.* 2001, *932*, 94-102; discussion 102-105.

[18] Tondo, L.; Baldessarini, R.J.; Hennen, J.; Minnai, G.P.; Salis, P.; Scamonatti, L.; Masia, M.; Ghiani, C.; Mannu, P. Suicide attempts in major affective disorder patients with comorbid substance use disorders. *J. Clin. Psychiatry.* 1999, *60 Suppl 2*, 63-69; discussion 75-66, 113-116.

[19] Tondo, L.; Lepri, B.; Baldessarini, R.J. Suicidal risks among 2826 Sardinian major affective disorder patients. *Acta Psychiatr. Scand.* 2007, *116*, 419-428.

[20] Judd, L.L.; Akiskal, H.S.; Schettler, P.J.; Endicott, J.; Maser, J.; Solomon, D.A.; Leon, A.C.; Rice, J.A.; Keller, M.B. The long-term natural history of the weekly symptomatic status of bipolar I disorder. *Arch. Gen. Psychiatry.* 2002, *59*, 530-537.

[21] Post, R.M.; Denicoff, K.D.; Leverich, G.S.; Altshuler, L.L.; Frye, M.A.; Suppes, T.M.; Rush, A.J.; Keck, P.E., Jr.; McElroy, S.L.; Luckenbaugh, D.A.; Pollio, C.; Kupka, R.; Nolen, W.A. Morbidity in 258 bipolar outpatients followed for 1 year with daily prospective ratings on the NIMH life chart method. *J. Clin. Psychiatry.* 2003, *64*, 680-690; quiz 738-689.

[22] Baldessarini, R.J.; Salvatore, P.; Tohen, M.; Khalsa, H.M.K.; Hennen, J.; González-Pinto, A.; Baethge, C.; Tohen, M. Morbidity from onset in first-episode bipolar I disorder patients: the International-300 study. *Neuropsychopharmacology*. 2004, *29*, S88.

[23] Joffe, R.T.; MacQueen, G.M.; Marriott, M.; Trevor Young, L. A prospective, longitudinal study of percentage of time spent ill in patients with bipolar I or bipolar II disorders. *Bipolar. Disord.* 2004, *6*, 62-66.

[24] Ghaemi, S.N.; Hsu, D.J.; Soldani, F.; Goodwin, F.K. Antidepressants in bipolar disorder: the case for caution. *Bipolar. Disord.* 2003, *5*, 421-433.

[25] Baldessarini, R.J.; Leahy, L.; Arcona, S.; Gause, D.; Zhang, W.; Hennen, J. Patterns of psychotropic drug prescription for U.S. patients with diagnoses of bipolar disorders. *Psychiatr. Serv.* 2007, *58*, 85-91.

[26] Koukopoulos, A.; Koukopoulos, A. Agitated depression as a mixed state and the problem of melancholia. *Psychiatr. Clin. North Am.* 1999, *22*, 547-564.

[27] Akiskal, H.S.; Benazzi, F.; Perugi, G.; Rihmer, Z. Agitated "unipolar" depression re-conceptualized as a depressive mixed state: implications for the antidepressant-suicide controversy. *J. Affect. Disord.* 2005, *85*, 245-258.

[28] Maj, M.; Pirozzi, R.; Magliano, L.; Fiorillo, A.; Bartoli, L. Agitated "unipolar" major depression: prevalence, phenomenology, and outcome. *J. Clin. Psychiatry*. 2006, *67*, 712-719.

[29] Electroconvulsive therapy. National Institutes of Health Consensus Development Conference Statement. *Natl. Inst. Health Consens. Dev. Conf. Consens. Statement.* 1985, *5*, 8 p.

[30] Weiner, R.D., *Practice of Electroconvulsive Therapy: Recommendations for Treatment, Training, and Privileging. A Task Force Report of the American Psychiatric Association*; 2nd ed.; American Psychiatric Association: Washington, 2000.

[31] Oquendo, M.A.; Chaudhury, S.R.; Mann, J.J. Pharmacotherapy of suicidal behavior in bipolar disorder. *Arch. Suicide Res.* 2005, *9*, 237-250.

[32] Angst, J.; Sellaro, R.; Angst, F. Long-term outcome and mortality of treated vs. untreated bipolar and depressed patients: A preliminary report. *International Journal of Psychiatric Clinical Practice.* 1998, *2*, 115–119.

[33] Baldessarini, R.J.; Jamison, K.R. Effects of medical interventions on suicidal behavior. Summary and conclusions. *J. Clin. Psychiatry.* 1999, *60 Suppl 2*, 117-122.

[34] Meltzer, H.Y.; Baldessarini, R.J. Reducing the risk for suicide in schizophrenia and affective disorders. *J. Clin. Psychiatry.* 2003, *64*, 1122-1129.

[35] Baldessarini, R.J.; Tarazi, F.I. Drug therapy of depression and anxiety disorders, psychosis and mania. In *Goodman and Gilman's Pharmacological Basis of Therapeutics*; 11 ed.; Brunton, L. L.; Lazo, J. S.; Parker, K. L., Eds.; McGraw-Hill Press: New York, 2005; pp. 429–500.

[36] Baldessarini, R.J.; Pompili, M.; Tondo, L.; Tsapakis, E.; Soldani, F.; Faedda, G.L.; Hennen, J. Antidepressants and Suicidal Behavior: Are We Hurting Or Helping? *Clinical Neuropsychiatry.* 2005, *2*, 73-75.

[37] Baldessarini, R.J.; Pompili, M.; Tondo, L. Suicidal risk in antidepressant drug trials. *Arch. Gen. Psychiatry.* 2006, *63*, 246-248.

[38] Mann, J.J.; Emslie, G.; Baldessarini, R.J.; Beardslee, W.; Fawcett, J.A.; Goodwin, F.K.; Leon, A.C.; Meltzer, H.Y.; Ryan, N.D.; Shaffer, D.; Wagner, K.D. ACNP Task Force report on SSRIs and suicidal behavior in youth. *Neuropsychopharmacology.* 2006, *31*, 473-492.

[39] Healy, D. Did regulators fail over selective serotonin reuptake inhibitors? *BMJ.* 2006, *333*, 92-95.

[40] Klein, D.F. FDA post-marketing safety decisions. *J. Clin. Psychiatry.* 2006, *67*, 1305-1306.

[41] Moller, H.J. Evidence for beneficial effects of antidepressants on suicidality in depressive patients: a systematic review. *Eur. Arch. Psychiatry Clin. Neurosci.* 2006, *256*, 329-343.

[42] Hall, W.D. How have the SSRI antidepressants affected suicide risk? *Lancet.* 2006, *367*, 1959-1962.

[43] Moller, H.J.; Baldwin, D.S.; Goodwin, G.; Kasper, S.; Okasha, A.; Stein, D.J.; Tandon, R.; Versiani, M. Do SSRIs or antidepressants in general increase suicidality? WPA Section on Pharmacopsychiatry: consensus statement. *Eur. Arch. Psychiatry Clin. Neurosci.* 2008, *258 Suppl. 3*, 3-23.

[44] Fergusson, D.; Doucette, S.; Glass, K.C.; Shapiro, S.; Healy, D.; Hebert, P.; Hutton, B. Association between suicide attempts and selective serotonin reuptake inhibitors: systematic review of randomised controlled trials. *BMJ.* 2005, *330*, 396.

[45] Gunnell, D.; Saperia, J.; Ashby, D. Selective serotonin reuptake inhibitors (SSRIs) and suicide in adults: meta-analysis of drug company data from placebo controlled, randomised controlled trials submitted to the MHRA's safety review. *BMJ.* 2005, *330*, 385.

[46] Stone, M.; Laughren, T.; Jones, M.L.; Levenson, M.; Holland, P.C.; Hughes, A.; Hammad, T.A.; Temple, R.; Rochester, G. Risk of suicidality in clinical trials of antidepressants in adults: analysis of proprietary data submitted to US Food and Drug Administration. *BMJ.* 2009, *339*, b2880.

[47] Laughren, T.; Levin, R. Food and Drug Administration perspective on negative symptoms in schizophrenia as a target for a drug treatment claim. *Schizophr. Bull.* 2006, *32*, 220-222.

[48] Leon, A.C. The revised warning for antidepressants and suicidality: unveiling the black box of statistical analyses. *Am. J. Psychiatry.* 2007, *164*, 1786-1789.

[49] Barbui, C.; Furukawa, T.A.; Cipriani, A. Effectiveness of paroxetine in the treatment of acute major depression in adults: a systematic re-examination of published and unpublished data from randomized trials. *Cmaj.* 2008, *178*, 296-305.

[50] Barbui, C.; Esposito, E.; Cipriani, A. Selective serotonin reuptake inhibitors and risk of suicide: a systematic review of observational studies. *Cmaj.* 2009, *180*, 291-297.

[51] Olfson, M.; Marcus, S.C.; Shaffer, D. Antidepressant drug therapy and suicide in severely depressed children and adults: A case-control study. *Arch. Gen. Psychiatry.* 2006, *63*, 865-872.

[52] Tiihonen, J.; Lonnqvist, J.; Wahlbeck, K.; Klaukka, T.; Tanskanen, A.; Haukka, J. Antidepressants and the risk of suicide, attempted suicide, and overall mortality in a nationwide cohort. *Arch. Gen. Psychiatry.* 2006, *63*, 1358-1367.

[53] Rahme, E.; Dasgupta, K.; Turecki, G.; Nedjar, H.; Galbaud du Fort, G. Risks of suicide and poisoning among elderly patients prescribed selective serotonin reuptake inhibitors: a retrospective cohort study. *J. Clin. Psychiatry.* 2008, *69*, 349-357.

[54] Cipriani, A.; Geddes, J.R.; Barbui, C. Venlafaxine for major depression. *BMJ.* 2007, *334*, 215-216.

[55] Dubicka, B.; Wilkinson, P. Evidence-based treatment of adolescent major depression. *Evid. Based Ment. Health.* 2007, *10*, 100-102.

[56] Helgason, T.; Tomasson, H.; Zoega, T. Antidepressants and public health in Iceland. Time series analysis of national data. *Br. J Psychiatry.* 2004, *184*, 157-162.

[57] Gibbons, R.D.; Hur, K.; Bhaumik, D.K.; Mann, J.J. The relationship between antidepressant medication use and rate of suicide. *Arch. Gen. Psychiatry.* 2005, *62*, 165-172.

[58] Gibbons, R.D.; Hur, K.; Bhaumik, D.K.; Mann, J.J. The relationship between antidepressant prescription rates and rate of early adolescent suicide. *Am. J. Psychiatry*. 2006, *163*, 1898-1904.

[59] Ludwig, J.; Marcotte, D.E. Anti-depressants, suicide, and drug regulation. *J. Policy Anal. Manage.* 2005, *24*, 249-272.

[60] Henriksson, S.; Isacsson, G. Increased antidepressant use and fewer suicides in Jamtland county, Sweden, after a primary care educational programme on the treatment of depression. *Acta Psychiatr. Scand.* 2006, *114*, 159-167.

[61] Isacsson, G.; Holmgren, P.; Ahlner, J. Selective serotonin reuptake inhibitor antidepressants and the risk of suicide: a controlled forensic database study of 14,857 suicides. *Acta Psychiatr. Scand* .2005, *111*, 286-290.

[62] Sondergard, L.; Kvist, K.; Lopez, A.G.; Andersen, P.K.; Kessing, L.V. Temporal changes in suicide rates for persons treated and not treated with antidepressants in Denmark during 1995-1999. *Acta Psychiatr. Scand.* 2006, *114*, 168-176.

[63] Reseland, S.; Bray, I.; Gunnell, D. Relationship between antidepressant sales and secular trends in suicide rates in the Nordic countries. *British Journal of Psychiatry. Vol.* 2006, *188*, 354-358.

[64] Freedman, D. The Ecological Fallacy. Available online: http://www.stat.berkeley.edu/~census/ecofall.txt (January, 10).

[65] Bailly, D. [Antidepressant use in children and adolescents]. *Arch. Pediatr.* 2009, *16*, 1415-1418.

[66] Alderman, C.P. Suicidal behavior and psychotropic medications for adolescents: an uneasy association, as yet not clarified. *Ann. Pharmacother.* 2009, *43*, 2093-2095.

[67] Masi, G.; Liboni, F.; Brovedani, P. Pharmacotherapy of major depressive disorder in adolescents. *Expert. Opin. Pharmacother.* 2010, *11*, 375-386.

[68] Schneeweiss, S.; Patrick, A.R.; Solomon, D.H.; Dormuth, C.R.; Miller, M.; Mehta, J.; Lee, J.C.; Wang, P.S. Comparative safety of antidepressant agents for children and adolescents regarding suicidal acts. *Pediatrics. 125*, 876-888.

[69] Reeves, R.R.; Ladner, M.E. Antidepressant-Induced Suicidality: An Update. *CNS Neurosci. Ther.* 2010.

[70] Jick, S.S.; Dean, A.D.; Jick, H. Antidepressants and suicide. *BMJ.* 1995, *310*, 215-218.

[71] Jick, H.; Kaye, J.A.; Jick, S.S. Antidepressants and the risk of suicidal behaviors. *JAMA*. 2004, *292*, 338-343.

[72] Warshaw, M.G.; Keller, M.B. The relationship between fluoxetine use and suicidal behavior in 654 subjects with anxiety disorders. *J. Clin. Psychiatry*. 1996, *57*, 158-166.

[73] Leon, A.C.; Keller, M.B.; Warshaw, M.G.; Mueller, T.I.; Soloman, D.A.; Coryell, W.; Endicott, J. A prospective study of fluoxetine treatment and suicidal behavior in affectively ill subjects. *Am. J. Psychiatry*. 1999, *156*, 195-201.

[74] Oquendo, M.A.; Kamali, M.; Ellis, S.P.; Grunebaum, M.F.; Malone, K.M.; Brodsky, B.S.; Sackeim, H.A.; Mann, J.J. Adequacy of antidepressant treatment after discharge and the occurrence of suicidal acts in major depression: A prospective study. *Am. J. Psychiatry*. 2002, *159*, 1746-1751.

[75] Yerevanian, B.I.; Koek, R.J.; Feusner, J.D.; Hwang, S.; Mintz, J. Antidepressants and suicidal behaviour in unipolar depression. *Acta Psychiatr. Scand.* 2004, *110*, 452-458.

[76] Angst, J.; Angst, F.; Gerber-Werder, R.; Gamma, A. Suicide in 406 mood-disorder patients with and without long-term medication: a 40 to 44 years' follow-up. *Arch. Suicide Res.* 2005, *9*, 279-300.

[77] Barak, Y.; Olmer, A.; Aizenberg, D. Antidepressants reduce the risk of suicide among elderly depressed patients. *Neuropsychopharmacology*. 2006, *31*, 178-181.

[78] Didham, R.C.; McConnell, D.W.; Blair, H.J.; Reith, D.M. Suicide and self-harm following prescription of SSRIs and other antidepressants: confounding by indication. *Br. J. Clin. Pharmacol.* 2005, *60*, 519-525.

[79] Martinez, C.; Rietbrock, S.; Wise, L.; Ashby, D.; Chick, J.; Moseley, J.; Evans, S.; Gunnell, D. Antidepressant treatment and the risk of fatal and non-fatal self harm in first episode depression: nested case-control study. *BMJ*. 2005, *330*, 389.

[80] Bauer, M.S.; Wisniewski, S.R.; Marangell, L.B.; Chessick, C.A.; Allen, M.H.; Dennehy, E.B.; Miklowitz, D.J.; Thase, M.E.; Sachs, G.S. Are antidepressants associated with new-onset suicidality in bipolar disorder? A prospective study of participants in the Systematic Treatment Enhancement Program for Bipolar Disorder (STEP-BD). *J. Clin. Psychiatry*. 2006, *67*, 48-55.

[81] Juurlink, D.N.; Mamdani, M.M.; Kopp, A.; Redelmeier, D.A. The risk of suicide with selective serotonin reuptake inhibitors in the elderly. *Am. J. Psychiatry*. 2006, *163*, 813-821.

[82] Simon, G.E.; Savarino, J.; Operskalski, B.; Wang, P.S. Suicide risk during antidepressant treatment. *Am. J. Psychiatry.* 2006, *163*, 41-47.
[83] Sondergard, L.; Kvist, K.; Andersen, P.K.; Kessing, L.V. Do antidepressants prevent suicide? *Int. Clin. Psychopharmacol.* 2006, *21*, 211-218.
[84] Sondergard, L.; Kvist, K.; Andersen, P.K.; Kessing, L.V. Do antidepressants precipitate youth suicide?: a nationwide pharmacoepidemiological study. *Eur. Child Adolesc. Psychiatry.* 2006, *15*, 232-240.
[85] Khan, A.; Warner, H.A.; Brown, W.A. Symptom reduction and suicide risk in patients treated with placebo in antidepressant clinical trials: an analysis of the Food and Drug Administration database. *Arch. Gen. Psychiatry.* 2000, *57*, 311-317.
[86] Khan, A.; Khan, S.; Kolts, R.; Brown, W.A. Suicide rates in clinical trials of SSRIs, other antidepressants, and placebo: analysis of FDA reports. *Am. J. Psychiatry.* 2003, *160*, 790-792.
[87] Acharya, N.; Rosen, A.S.; Polzer, J.P.; D'Souza, D.N.; Perahia, D.G.; Cavazzoni, P.A.; Baldessarini, R.J. Duloxetine: meta-analyses of suicidal behaviors and ideation in clinical trials for major depressive disorder. *J. Clin. Psychopharmacol.* 2006, *26*, 587-594.
[88] Bostwick, J.M.; Pankratz, V.S. Affective disorders and suicide risk: a reexamination. *Am. J. Psychiatry.* 2000, *157*, 1925-1932.
[89] Tollefson, G.D.; Rampey, A.H., Jr.; Beasley, C.M., Jr.; Enas, G.G.; Potvin, J.H. Absence of a relationship between adverse events and suicidality during pharmacotherapy for depression. *J. Clin. Psychopharmacol.* 1994, *14*, 163-169.
[90] Storosum, J.G.; van Zwieten, B.J.; van den Brink, W.; Gersons, B.P.; Broekmans, A.W. Suicide risk in placebo-controlled studies of major depression. *Am. J. Psychiatry.* 2001, *158*, 1271-1275.
[91] U.S. Food and Drug Administration (FDA) Antidepressant use in children, adolescents, and adults. Available online: http://www.fda.gov/Drugs/DrugSafety/InformationbyDrugClass/UCM096273 (June 1).
[92] Hammad, T.A.; Laughren, T.P.; Racoosin, J.A. Suicide rates in short-term randomized controlled trials of newer antidepressants. *J. Clin. Psychopharmacol.* 2006, *26*, 203-207.
[93] Hammad, T.A.; Laughren, T.; Racoosin, J. Suicidality in pediatric patients treated with antidepressant drugs. *Arch. Gen. Psychiatry.* 2006, *63*, 332-339.

[94] MHRA (UK Medicines and Health Regulatory Agency) Selective serotonin reuptake inhibitor (SSRI) antidepressants: Committee on Safety of Medicines (CSM) working group findings. Available online: http://www.mhra.gov.uk/news/2004/2004.htm (September, 22).

[95] Beasley, C.M., Jr.; Dornseif, B.E.; Bosomworth, J.C.; Sayler, M.E.; Rampey, A.H., Jr.; Heiligenstein, J.H.; Thompson, V.L.; Murphy, D.J.; Masica, D.N. Fluoxetine and suicide: a meta-analysis of controlled trials of treatment for depression. *BMJ.* 1991, *303*, 685-692.

[96] Filteau, M.J.; Lapierre, Y.D.; Bakish, D.; Blanchard, A. Reduction in suicidal ideation with SSRIs: a review of 459 depressed patients. *J. Psychiatry Neurosci.* 1993, *18*, 114-119.

[97] Pedersen, A.G. Escitalopram and suicidality in adult depression and anxiety. *Int. Clin. Psychopharmacol.* 2005, *20*, 139-143.

[98] Baldessarini, R.J.; Tondo, L. Psychopharmacology for suicide prevention. In *Suicide in psichiatric disorders*; Tatarelli, R.; Pompili, M.; Girardi, P., Eds.; Nova Science Publischers Inc.: New York, 2007.

[99] Tsapakis, E.M.; Soldani, F.; Tondo, L.; Baldessarini, R.J. Efficacy of antidepressants in juvenile depression: meta-analysis. *Br. J. Psychiatry.* 2008, *193*, 10-17.

[100] March, J.; Silva, S.; Petrycki, S.; Curry, J.; Wells, K.; Fairbank, J.; Burns, B.; Domino, M.; McNulty, S.; Vitiello, B.; Severe, J. Fluoxetine, cognitive-behavioral therapy, and their combination for adolescents with depression: Treatment for Adolescents With Depression Study (TADS) randomized controlled trial. *JAMA.* 2004, *292*, 807-820.

[101] Barbui, C.; Campomori, A.; D'Avanzo, B.; Negri, E.; Garattini, S. Antidepressant drug use in Italy since the introduction of SSRIs: national trends, regional differences and impact on suicide rates. *Soc. Psychiatry Psychiatr. Epidemiol.* 1999, *34*, 152-156.

[102] Guaiana, G.; Andretta, M.; Corbari, L.; Mirandola, M.; Sorio, A.; D'Avanzo, B.; Barbui, C. Antidepressant drug consumption and public health indicators in Italy, 1955 to 2000. *J. Clin. Psychiatry.* 2005, *66*, 750-755.

[103] Carlsten, A.; Waern, M.; Ekedahl, A.; Ranstam, J. Antidepressant medication and suicide in Sweden. *Pharmacoepidemiol. Drug Saf.* 2001, *10*, 525-530.

[104] Ohberg, A.; Vuori, E.; Klaukka, T.; Lonnqvist, J. Antidepressants and suicide mortality. *J. Affect. Disord.* 1998, *50*, 225-233.

[105] Rihmer, Z.; Appleby, L.; Rihmer, A.; Belso, N. Decreasing suicide in Hungary. *Br. J. Psychiatry.* 2000, *177*, 84.

[106] Rihmer, Z. Can better recognition and treatment of depression reduce suicide rates? A brief review. *Eur. Psychiatry.* 2001, *16*, 406-409.

[107] Rihmer, Z. Do SSRIs increase the risk of suicide among depressives even if they are taking only placebo? *Psychother. Psychosom.* 2003, *72*, 357-358; author reply 359-360.

[108] Hall, W.D.; Mant, A.; Mitchell, P.B.; Rendle, V.A.; Hickie, I.B.; McManus, P. Association between antidepressant prescribing and suicide in Australia, 1991-2000: trend analysis. *BMJ.* 2003, *326*, 1008.

[109] Levi, F.; La Vecchia, C.; Lucchini, F.; Negri, E.; Saxena, S.; Maulik, P.K.; Saraceno, B. Trends in mortality from suicide, 1965-99. *Acta Psychiatr. Scand.* 2003, *108*, 341-349.

[110] Levi, F.; La Vecchia, C.; Saraceno, B. Global suicide rates. *Eur. J. Public Health.* 2003, *13*, 97-98.

[111] Davis, A.; Gilhooley, M.; Agius, M.; Zaman, R. Suicide risk and choice of antidepressant. *Psychiatr. Danub.* 2010, *22*, 358-359.

[112] Gunnell, D.; Middleton, N.; Whitley, E.; Dorling, D.; Frankel, S. Why are suicide rates rising in young men but falling in the elderly?-- a time-series analysis of trends in England and Wales 1950-1998. *Soc. Sci. Med.* 2003, *57*, 595-611.

[113] Kasper, S.; Montgomery, S.A.; Moller, H.J.; van Oers, H.J.; Jan Schutte, A.; Vrijland, P.; van der Meulen, E.A. Longitudinal analysis of the suicidal behaviour risk in short-term placebo-controlled studies of mirtazapine in major depressive disorder. *World J. Biol. Psychiatry.* 2010, *11*, 36-44.

[114] Kelly, C.B.; Ansari, T.; Rafferty, T.; Stevenson, M. Antidepressant prescribing and suicide rate in Northern Ireland. *Eur. Psychiatry.* 2003, *18*, 325-328.

[115] Gunnell, D.; Ashby, D. Antidepressants and suicide: what is the balance of benefit and harm. *BMJ.* 2004, *329*, 34-38.

[116] Morgan, O.W.; Griffiths, C.; Majeed, A. Association between mortality from suicide in England and antidepressant prescribing: an ecological study. *BMC Public Health.* 2004, *4*, 63.

[117] Barak, Y.; Aizenberg, D. Association between antidepressant prescribing and suicide in Israel. *Int. Clin. Psychopharmacol.* 2006, *21*, 281-284.

[118] Matthews, J.D.; Fava, M. Risk of suicidality in depression with serotonergic antidepressants. *Ann. Clin. Psychiatry.* 2000, *12*, 43-50.

[119] Baldessarini, R.J.; Willmuth, R.L. Psychotic reactions during amitriptyline therapy. *Can. Psychiatr. Assoc. J.* 1968, *13*, 571-573.

[120] Teicher, M.H.; Glod, C.; Cole, J.O. Emergence of intense suicidal preoccupation during fluoxetine treatment. *Am. J. Psychiatry.* 1990, *147*, 207-210.

[121] Teicher, M.H.; Glod, C.A.; Cole, J.O. Antidepressant drugs and the emergence of suicidal tendencies. *Drug Saf.* 1993, *8*, 186-212.

[122] Damluji, N.F.; Ferguson, J.M. Paradoxical worsening of depressive symptomatology caused by antidepressants. *J. Clin. Psychopharmacol.* 1988, *8*, 347-349.

[123] Healy, D.; Whitaker, C. Antidepressants and suicide: risk-benefit conundrums. *J. Psychiatry Neurosci.* 2003, *28*, 331-337.

[124] Whittington, C.J.; Kendall, T.; Fonagy, P.; Cottrell, D.; Cotgrove, A.; Boddington, E. Selective serotonin reuptake inhibitors in childhood depression: systematic review of published versus unpublished data. *Lancet.* 2004, *363*, 1341-1345.

[125] Jureidini, J.N.; Doecke, C.J.; Mansfield, P.R.; Haby, M.M.; Menkes, D.B.; Tonkin, A.L. Efficacy and safety of antidepressants for children and adolescents. *BMJ.* 2004, *328*, 879-883.

[126] Herxheimer, A.; Mintzes, B. Antidepressants and adverse effects in young patients: uncovering the evidence. *Cmaj.* 2004, *170*, 487-489.

[127] Barbui, C. Antidepressants and the risk of suicidal behaviors. *Jama.* 2004, *292*, 2833; author reply 2833.

[128] Valuck, R.J.; Libby, A.M.; Sills, M.R.; Giese, A.A.; Allen, R.R. Antidepressant treatment and risk of suicide attempt by adolescents with major depressive disorder: a propensity-adjusted retrospective cohort study. *CNS Drugs.* 2004, *18*, 1119-1132.

[129] Rubino, A.; Roskell, N.; Tennis, P.; Mines, D.; Weich, S.; Andrews, E. Risk of suicide during treatment with venlafaxine, citalopram, fluoxetine, and dothiepin: retrospective cohort study. *BMJ.* 2007, *334*, 242.

[130] Pompili, M.; Tondo, L.; Baldessarini, R.J. Suicidal Risk Emerging During Antidepressant Treatment: Recognition and Intervention. *Clinical Neuropsychiatry.* 2005, *2*, 66-72.

Index

N

O

P

R

S

T